I0505166

My Hormones Are Killing Me:

Living with Adenomyosis and Estrogen Dominance

Maria Yeager

©Copyright 2012 Maria Yeager
All rights reserved

No part of this book may be reproduced or transmitted in any form or by any means, electronic or mechanical, including photocopying, recording, or by any information storage and retrieval system, without the written permission of the author and except where permitted by law.

ISBN-13:
978-1508714989

ISBN-10:
1508714983

Printed in the United States of America

Cover design by Victor Rook – author, filmmaker, photographer, and web designer. His nature film *Beyond the Garden Gate* ran on PBS for four years and is the winner of two Telly Awards.

Note: Names of the physicians involved in the 17-year course of treatment discussed in this book have been changed to protect the individual's identity. Any similarity in name to any active or retired physician is purely coincidental.

Table of Contents

Introduction

Adenomyosis....this is a word I had never heard of until just a few years ago. Most of my life I had heard about fibroids, endometriosis, painful cramps, heavy bleeding - all associated with a woman's menstrual cycle - but adenomyosis was a term that didn't come up until I was in my forties. I wondered why I had not heard about this little known disorder of the uterus during my seventeen year journey of severe pain and heavy bleeding.

My story began in 1990 with my first attack of severe abdominal pain. For the next seventeen years, I had numerous medical tests, surgeries and procedures performed to find the cause of my pain. I was also put on a list of medications that could fill up this entire page. The list of doctors that I saw during this period is probably just as long as my medication list. I did not get complete relief from my pain until my hysterectomy in 2007. It was at that time that I learned I had been suffering from adenomyosis.

I decided to do some research and learned quite a bit about this disorder. I learned that this condition is very difficult to diagnose, and it can't be definitively diagnosed without doing a hysterectomy. I was so discouraged when I learned this. I thought about all the other people out there who might be suffering with the same condition. I can empathize with the frustration of not being able to get any pain relief because of a lack of a solid diagnosis. As I continued my research, this book took on a life of its own. Through my research, I learned that adenomyosis has been linked to a condition called estrogen dominance. As I learned more about this condition, all the pieces of my medical history suddenly came into clear focus. When I realized that a simple hormonal imbalance could cause a myriad of health conditions, I became even more motivated to get this information out to the general public.

I am writing this book to help those out who might be suffering from similar symptoms. I strongly believe that more attention and research need to be given to not only adenomyosis but also the possible underlying condition of estrogen dominance. It is also very important to get this information out there so others may get help quicker than I received my diagnosis. Even if I just help one person, writing this book will be worth the effort.

The Early Years

Growing up in a small suburb of Cincinnati, Ohio, I had very few health problems. Of course I had the occasional cold or flu, but other than that, I was a fairly healthy, active and happy child. My menstrual cycles started when I was 14 years old which is normal by any measure. However, as my teen years progressed, I noticed that my periods were quite painful, lasting up to ten days, and were very heavy. There were times during those years when I was having so much pain that I could barely walk. I was given NSAIDS to help control the pain from the cramps. This did help some, but I remember thinking that I seemed to have more problems with my cycle than my other friends.

My family did have a history of some health issues involving the reproductive organs. My maternal grandmother was diagnosed with breast cancer in her late 30's, and she passed away from this disease in 1940 at age 41. I have been told she also suffered terribly from asthma and severe allergies. Stories have been told about how family members would take her on vacation to Michigan to get some relief when her allergies were at their worst. Later in life, her sister also died of breast cancer. In addition to my maternal grandmother's health issues, other family members have suffered from heavy and painful menstruation, passing large blood clots during menstruation, uterine fibroid tumors and even osteopenia during the premenopausal years. When I started having trouble, I didn't think too much about it because a lot of my family members endured similar symptoms.

I specifically remember having horrible cramping and very heavy bleeding one summer day during my teen years. Some of my friends wanted to go to a movie, and I really wanted to go. I took Motrin during the morning hoping that it would help the cramping in time for me to be able to go to the movie. I curled up in a fetal position on the couch and waited for the cramps to pass. The cramps were intense, and I was sweating and felt nauseated. I was so pale that I looked like a ghost! When it came time to go to the movie, I decided to go even though I felt awful. For the first half of the show, I was in such pain that I really didn't enjoy myself at all, but the cramps finally started to let up about halfway through the movie. By the time I left, I wasn't in too much pain, but I was utterly exhausted. I slept like a log that night.

In 1983, I left home to attend Eastern Kentucky University. I continued to have very heavy periods and some pretty intense cramping.

Living in a dorm with a bunch of women made me realize that I wasn't alone in dealing with menstrual issues. Some of them had horrible pain and looked terrible during that time, and others just seemed to get through each month like it was nothing at all. I was so jealous of those lucky girls who had it easy each month! Seeing this, I came to the realization that I was just one of those unlucky girls who gets to go through life with long, heavy and painful periods. But, I wasn't the only one!

Around this same time, I began to suffer terribly from allergies. I remember being in class at EKU trying desperately to listen to my professor while holding a Kleenex up to my nose due to the terrible congestion. I would hold that Kleenex with one hand and try and take notes with the other hand. It was miserable, but I just accepted it thinking that this was just some kind of genetic thing since my family had a strong history of allergies, especially on my mom's side.

Then, in the summer of 1985 while on summer break from college, I woke up one night with tremendous abdominal pain and nausea. I had just worked a ten hour shift the day before, and I felt fine during work. Luckily, I was at home and not at school when this happened. I thought I had the stomach flu at first, but the abdominal pain became so severe that I began to think that something much worse was happening to me. I vomited for several hours, and then I started to have dry heaves. The abdominal pain was intense. I tried to sleep but would wake up and realize that I had only been asleep for a few minutes. When the dry heaving finally slowed down, my mom made me some soup and tried to get me to eat some of it. I tried, but it was almost as if there was something in my throat preventing me from swallowing. I absolutely could not swallow one sip of soup. I gave up and went to rest on the couch. I slept about 45 minutes, the most I had slept in about 24 hours, but when I woke up, I had such severe abdominal pain that I could barely stand up. My mom decided to call the doctor, and he told her to give me some Mylanta. He said that if she didn't notice improvement in me over the next few hours to take me to the emergency room. Finally that evening, my mom decided enough was enough, and she drove me to the hospital. As I look back on it now, I have spotty memories of what happened from this point forward. The only memory that I remember of my trip to the hospital was holding a pillow to my stomach and looking up at my mom as she was driving. I must have been blacking out as I had to rely on my mom's recollection of what happened from this point forward.

We arrived at the hospital, and I was taken back for the examination. The emergency room doctor believed that I had a bad case of the stomach flu. I was severely dehydrated, so I was put on an IV for rehydration. I was given some kind of milky drink that was supposed to settle my stomach, but about 15 minutes after drinking it, I vomited it up. After this, I can only recall a few moments until the following day. I found out later that the doctor had ordered some sleep medication to be put into my IV, so I had been sedated. When I had finished receiving fluids through the IV, the emergency room doctor once again came in and was very concerned about my condition. He decided to examine me one more time before I left to go home. This time, he pressed on the right side of my abdomen, and I jumped. Seeing this, he immediately ordered a complete blood count. When the test came back, I think everyone was shocked. I had an extremely high white blood cell count that, coupled with the right sided abdominal pain, suggested appendicitis. He called my uncle who was a surgeon to come in to perform an appendectomy.

I remember my uncle standing over top of me and talking to me.

"Maria, you have acute appendicitis, and we have to operate."

"When?" I asked.

"Right now" he replied.

That was about 2 a.m. I was wheeled into surgery at around 3 a.m.

When I woke up from surgery, I was shocked to find out that I did indeed have appendicitis. In fact, the appendix had ruptured and was covered with gangrene. My uncle told my mom that it was probably the worst appendix he had ever seen! He said I was going to be sick for a very long time.

The next morning, I remember being visited by nurses from other floors and even the pathologist who examined my ruptured appendix. They were amazed that I actually walked into the hospital the previous night.

"You should have been come in here by ambulance and unconscious! How in the world did you walk in here with an appendix in that kind of shape?"

Nurses, lab workers and even my uncle were so surprised that I was able to walk into the hospital on my own accord. The pathologist said that it was the worst appendix that he had ever examined in his lab.

I recovered quicker than most people expected. In fact, I was back to work three weeks after surgery. I vividly remember the horrible abdominal pain associated with this ruptured appendix, and I will never forget what my uncle said to me:

> "Maria, if you EVER have pain like that again, get yourself to a hospital IMMEDIATELY! This could have killed you!"

This one statement stayed with me and ended up playing a major role in what I was about to go through....

The First Full Blown Attack

16

Three years after graduating from college, I was working at a laboratory in South Carolina. It was a Friday night in the spring of 1990, and I was going on a date with my boyfriend at the time. I was really looking forward to this as it had been a really busy week for me. I felt great, and we went out to eat and to a movie. After the date, I went home and went to bed. My period was just ending, and I was feeling a little tired.

At about 4 a.m., I woke up to extremely bad abdominal pain and nausea. I had not felt this sick since my ruptured appendix. I couldn't stand up because of the pain, and I literally crawled to the bathroom. The pain was coming in waves across my lower abdomen and into the small of my back. Sweat was dripping down the sides of my face and I felt extremely nauseated. I pushed myself up on the toilet because I felt like I had to have a bowel movement. However, I couldn't. The waves of pain kept coming over me, and at times I felt like I was going to faint. My whole shirt and my hair were wet with sweat. I would put my hands on the sink and bend over and just try to breathe through the waves of pain. A couple of times, I got so lightheaded I saw stars. I kept telling myself that I couldn't pass out because I was alone in that apartment. Thinking back on what happened when I had a ruptured appendix, I began to panic, thinking that something terrible was happening to me. Was this somehow linked to the appendicitis? All I could think about was that statement from my uncle,

> "Maria, if you EVER have pain like that again, get yourself to a hospital IMMEDIATELY! This could have killed you!"

What was happening? Should I go to the hospital now or give it some time? Being a scientist, the thought crossed my mind that this was a complication of the ruptured appendix. Did I have an intestinal obstruction? This pain was so severe, and waiting might be a terrible decision, especially after what my uncle told me. I was terrified! Finally I called my mom. She immediately came over to take me to the hospital. While I was waiting on her, I started to think about how I was going to let her in. I was in so much pain that I didn't think I was going to be able to make it to the front door of my apartment. When the doorbell rang, somehow I mustered up every bit of strength that I had to get to that door.

> "What happened?" she asked.

"I don't know. All I know is I'm in severe pain and I don't think I can make it to the car," I replied. I was scared stiff, and all I could think of was what had happened to me when my appendix had ruptured.

"You can do it. Come on. You can make it."

She grabbed hold of me, and I put my arm around her. Although I was doubled over in pain, I did make it to the car. She drove to the hospital, and all I could do was to try to stay calm and just breathe.

When we arrived, my mom helped me into the emergency room. My mom filled out all the paperwork while I sat there doubled over in pain. Then suddenly I had the urge to go to the bathroom. I rushed to the restroom, and this time I had a severe case of diarrhea. I went back to the waiting room noticing that I had a little bit of pain relief. A few minutes later, I was called back to see the doctor.

When the doctor came in, I was lying on the stretcher in the fetal position. Although I did get a little bit of relief after the bout of diarrhea, the pain was still so severe that I could not lie flat. He examined me and ran some tests and concluded that I probably had a case of food poisoning. He gave me a shot for the pain and told us to come back if my condition worsened. So I went home and slept the rest of the day as a result of the pain shot that I had been given.

The next day I felt fine except for being just a little bit tired. I drank lots of fluids and assumed this was just the stomach flu. I rested for a few days and then returned to my normal schedule. I thought that this was just a one time thing and that it would probably never happen again. I could not have been more wrong.

The "Valley"

I refer to the years between 1992 and 1998 as "the valley" because I was having attacks of severe abdominal pain, sometimes as many as once a month. Both my social and work life were affected during this time. I suffered not only physically but also emotionally as I had severe depression. It is because of this difficult time that I am writing this book. I want people to be aware of this disorder and the kind of toll it can take on the person who has to deal with it.

About a year after the first attack, I was asleep once again when I awoke to the same severe and debilitating pain that had attacked me on that fateful Friday night in 1990. Once again, this was right at the end of my period. The pain was unbearable, and again I was cramping in my abdomen with the pain moving into the small of my back. I crawled to the bathroom and laid there in the fetal position and began to cry. Sweat was dripping down my face and my shirt was soaked. Every time I tried to stand up, I felt like I was going to pass out.

"What is this??? Why is this happening to me again?"

While fighting through the pain, I was feeling angry, confused, sad and frustrated. It was a horrible night.

I kept trying to go to the bathroom but I couldn't. I felt this horrendous need to push. In fact, I started to wonder if I was having a miscarriage. The pain kept coming in waves, and all I felt this was worse than the ruptured appendix. I was convinced that something serious was going on, and the doctor at the hospital missed it the first time. Eventually, I had another bout of diarrhea, and the pain eventually subsided. I decided to make an appointment the next day to see a family doctor instead of making another trip to the emergency room.

The next day, I went to see Dr. Jones who was a family practitioner. I explained that this was the second episode of severe abdominal pain in the past two years. We reviewed in detail the symptoms that I had been experiencing, and I made sure to tell him that both episodes occurred at the very end of my period. He felt like this was just another episode of food poisoning, but he did mention the possibility that I might be suffering from irritable bowel syndrome. I was sent home with no definitive diagnosis and was told to come back if the pain returned.

After this second episode, the attacks started to become more frequent. I began to recognize that the attacks always happened at the same time each month - right at the end of my period. I also started to notice that right before an attack my stomach would swell, and at times I looked like I was pregnant. I was convinced that this was somehow related to my menstrual cycle. I was becoming more and more concerned that I might be having a miscarriage during these attacks. Additionally, I noticed that the pain seemed to affect my left side more than my right side. The next appointment that I made was with a gynecologist.

I was very happy to go to my first appointment with Dr. Kennedy. Since I had been noticing that these symptoms were occurring around the time of my menstrual cycle, I was sure that the gynecologist would have an answer for what was causing all of this pain. I had a lot of faith in doctors back then and I expected to leave the office that day with an answer and an effective treatment.

But to my disappointment, Dr. Kennedy wasn't sure what was going on either. He explained to me that I should start taking Motrin several days before the start of my period and continue taking it until the end of my period. He explained that the Motrin would block the prostaglandins in my body that were the culprits in the pain associated with menstrual cramps. I left pretty upset because I thought that all he did was give me pain medication but didn't get to the root cause of the problem. I told my co-workers what the doctor had said, and they were disgusted. Just a pain reliever? Really? Only later did I realize that his thinking was closer to the root cause of the problem than I had thought!

The attacks continued. They became more severe and more frequent. I was starting to fall into a depression and was so anxious during the latter part of my period that I was almost afraid to leave my house. I was scared that an attack would happen when I wasn't close to a bathroom or out in public where I couldn't get home quickly. I returned a second time to Dr. Kennedy.

This time, he suggested that I start to take a birth control pill to help control the severe cramping pain. My husband and I wanted to have children so I wasn't too happy about the idea, but I realized I wasn't going to be able to function without taking them. I was hesitant but agreed to try this option. I began taking the birth control pill in April, 1998.

After being on the pill for only a couple of weeks, I started to bleed. The bleeding continued for about fifteen days before I decided to go back to the gynecologist once again.

"I've been bleeding for fifteen days straight and I'm not slowing down. What's going on?" I asked Dr. Kennedy.

"Well sometimes it takes several months for your body to adjust to the pill. Give it a couple more months to see if your body will adjust to it."

I agreed to do this, but during the next few months, I stopped for about two weeks and then bled for two weeks and so forth. This was driving me crazy and I really felt tired, probably because of all the blood loss. I returned once again to the gynecologist. This time he took me off that pill and switched me to another kind of birth control pill.

"Give it a couple of months. Hopefully this one will work."

I agreed once again to do this, but I was getting a little frustrated. During the first few months, I did have some irregular bleeding but it wasn't as bad as the first pill that he had prescribed. However, I began to have frequent yeast infections which continued through my reproductive years. For the next 15 years or so, I bought quite a few tubes of Monistat.

A few months later, I woke up to searing abdominal pain. This was the same cramping pain that came in waves as before. The pain was so severe that I would be on all fours just rocking back and forth and praying to God to get me through the cramp without passing out. Again my shirt was soaked and sweat was dripping off my face. My lower stomach was so bloated that anyone who saw me would have probably thought that I was pregnant. This time, the nausea was so bad that I threw up several times during the attack. After about three hours or so, the pain started to let up and I went back to bed. When I finally got up the next day, I was so exhausted and exasperated that I didn't know what to do. I finally decided to make another trip back to Dr. Jones.

"Something is seriously wrong. The pain that I am feeling with these attacks is actually worse than what I remember when I had a ruptured appendix. What else can we do to figure this out?" I asked.

"Well, this kind of sounds like irritable bowel syndrome. I think you need to go and see a gastroenterologist. I will refer you to a good one in this town."

I was so frustrated! Here I was, having severe abdominal pain that seemed to be worse than what I had with my ruptured appendix, and no one could give me a definitive diagnosis. I took a deep breath, and I tried to calm myself down. Maybe the problem was in my gastrointestinal tract. It was still kind of funny that the pain always seemed to come at the end of my menstrual cycle. But, at this point, I was willing to look at any possibility to end these attacks.

Dr. Hamilton was very personable and seemed genuinely concerned about me and all the pain that I had endured. His first thought was to do a colonoscopy to see if there was any abnormality in the large intestine. He was also particularly concerned about residual problems from my ruptured appendix such as a blockage in my intestine. I absolutely dreaded the thought of having this procedure done, but when you are in such pain, believe me, you will agree to do just about any medical test to find a solution.

A few weeks later, I began the prep for the colonoscopy. This involved drinking a very large container of medicated liquid which would make me go to the bathroom all night. This was the worst part of the colonoscopy experience. I had to drink 8 ounces of this liquid every twenty minutes until it was gone. First of all, it tasted like salt water. About halfway through the container, I started to go to the bathroom and went continuously through half of the night. Several hours into drinking this stuff, I got very cold and was walking around with a big blanket around me. When I got to the very bottom of the container, I became very nauseated and couldn't finish it.

The next morning, I went to the office to have the colonoscopy, and in addition to being nauseated, I was a nervous wreck. However, the colonoscopy itself wasn't bad at all. The doctor put me into a light sleep, and I don't remember a thing. When I woke up, I felt fine - no nausea and no pain. Dr. Hamilton came in and spoke to us and told us that I had a very healthy colon and that the appendix area was also fine. He could find no abnormality at all in the colon that would explain my episodes of pain. Although this should have been good news, I felt frustrated because I still did not have a reason for my episodes of severe abdominal pain. He gave me the antispasmodic drug Levsin to take during the attacks of pain. His opinion was that I may have been suffering from irritable bowel syndrome.

> *Levsin, also known as hyoscyamine, is an antispasmodic medication. It is primarily used in the treatment of stomach and bowel problems. Specifically, it has been used to treat irritable bowel syndrome, diverticulitis, peptic ulcers, pancreatitis, colitis, cystitis, bladder spasms, Parkinson's disease and rhinitis. Some of the side effects include drowsiness, dizziness, nervousness, weakness, headache, constipation, bloating, nausea, vomiting, dry mouth, blurry vision, fast heart rate, and rash.*

> *Irritable bowel syndrome refers to an intestinal disorder in which the process of peristalsis malfunctions. In other words, the squeezing action of the large intestine gets out of sync and causes abdominal pain, cramping and changes in bowel habits. This can result in constipation, diarrhea or alternating episodes of both. One in 6 people have IBS, and it is the number one reason a person goes to see a gastroenterologist. Diagnosis is made after exclusion of other more serious gastrointestinal disorders.*

Abdominal pain was not the only thing I was trying to deal with during this time. I was getting continual head infections, and I had been on and off antibiotics for months. Finally, a close friend of mine suggested that these "head infections" were actually allergies. That intrigued me, so I went to see an allergist. Sure enough, the allergy prick test showed that I had significant allergies, particularly to trees, grasses and ragweed. I began taking allergy shots and continued on these for years to come. Luckily, the shots did help me dramatically.

I continued to take the birth control pill and hoped that these attacks would eventually resolve. However, they did not. I was desperate and didn't know what to do. I was so depressed and anxious and didn't know where to turn at this point. I mentioned my problems to a friend who proceeded to tell me about a reproductive endocrinologist that she had been seeing because of severe PMS. She highly recommended Dr. Suri, but it would mean that I would have to travel one hour each way to see her since this doctor was not in the town where I lived. Desperate times call for desperate measures, so I decided to go to her irregardless of the amount of travel time to her office.

During my first appointment, I spent a long time with Dr. Suri explaining the symptoms and concerns that I had for the past several years. She did a thorough exam on me and suggested that I once again change to a different birth control pill. She basically explained to me that each pill has differing amounts of estrogen and progesterone, and it would take some time to see which pill would work for me. During the exam, everything appeared to be normal, but she said she would call me back with the results of my blood work. So, I went home with the birth control pill Orthocyclen, and I waited for the test results.

About a week later, the receptionist from Dr. Suri's office called me. All of the blood work, including a CBC and thyroid test, came back normal. I was advised to stay on the current birth control pill for several months to allow my body to adjust to it. If I had any further problems after that, I was told to call the office for a follow up appointment.

I waited about 6 months to see if the abnormal bleeding would correct itself; however, it did not improve. I was having very heavy menstrual bleeding that would last for about ten days, and I would have spotting in between each period. Additionally, I continued to have attacks of debilitating abdominal pain toward the end of my period. During some months the pain was extremely severe, and during other months the pain was just moderate. After this 6 month time period was over, I decided to make another appointment with Dr. Suri.

During this second appointment, we reviewed all my symptoms from the previous 6 months. She decided that it would be a good idea for me to undergo a dilation and curettage (D&C). I filled out all of the paperwork, had the necessary blood tests performed, and in November 1995, I entered the hospital ready to have the D&C.

All kinds of thoughts were racing through my head.

"How much pain will I be in when I wake up?"

"What if they find that if I have some kind of horrible disease?"
"Will I ever be able to have children? What if they have to remove my uterus?"
"What if they find cancer?"

Looking back on this now, I was worrying myself sick for no good reason. But at the time, I was really terrified.

I was taken back to the operating room and put to sleep. When I woke up, I was shaking uncontrollably. I remember the nurses covering me up with a bunch of warm blankets and hearing them talk about how much I was shaking. To this day, I don't know why I came out of surgery in that condition. When I finally was able to talk, I asked the nurses what Dr. Suri found during the surgery.

"Just dysfunctional uterine bleeding. Nothing serious. You are going to be just fine."

It was a bittersweet moment for me. On one hand, nothing serious was found, but on the other hand, what was causing this pain? No one seemed to be able to give me a straight answer. So, after staying in recovery for a few hours, we went home hoping that this procedure would at least reduce the amount of blood loss each month during my period.

My periods did become a little lighter after that, and the spotting in between the periods finally stopped. I stayed on Orthocyclen for several years after this, but I continued to have attacks of severe abdominal pain every couple of months.

During my next appointment with Dr. Suri, I explained to her that these abdominal pain attacks were continuing and were causing me a great deal of distress. At this point, she recommended to me that I have a laparoscopy to rule out any problem with the uterus or ovaries. During this surgery, she planned to take a look around the area of the appendix and see if there were any adhesions that may be causing some of the pain. We agreed to go ahead with this surgery.

All of those same questions were racing through my head -

"What if they find something serious?"

"What if I can't have children?"

"When am I going to get an answer and when is this all going to be over?"

During the operation, my doctor performed a tubal insufflation to make sure the fallopian tubes were open. She did this because we had been trying for a pregnancy ever since we got married in 1992 and hadn't had any luck. However, the tubes were found to be open without any kind of blockage that might be contributing to my infertility. Additionally, she found "slight" endometriosis on the right ovary and uterus, and these implants were ablated by laser.

During my follow up appointment with Dr. Suri, she reiterated that she did find some endometriosis on the ovaries and uterus. She explained that the degree of endometriosis did not determine the degree of pain that I was feeling. Apparently, some people with a great deal of endometrial implants have very little pain, and some people with very little endometriosis have severe pain. She showed me pictures that she took during the surgery. She noted that other than the few endometrial implants, the uterus and ovaries appeared normal. Her opinion was that the source of the pain was endometriosis.

Endometriosis is a condition where endometrial cells found inside the uterus that are shed each month in the form of a menstrual period are found outside of the uterus. Common sites of implants are the ovaries, bladder, bowel and rectum. Symptoms can include pelvic and lower back pain, infertility, irregular bleeding and pain with bowel movements.

The abdominal pains associated with my periods were really having a terrible impact on my mental health. I began to have what I now believe are panic attacks. If I was out in public and my stomach would start to swell or I felt a little bit of abdominal discomfort, my heart would start to race and I would get really dizzy. As soon as the first little symptom reared its ugly head, no matter where I was, I immediately would go home. Nausea would set in and I would get shaky, so much so that at times I would feel like I might faint. I was petrified that an attack would come over me and I wouldn't be close to home. I was in absolute misery, so I once again returned to Dr. Jones.

During this visit, the doctor diagnosed me with irritable bowel syndrome (IBS). I was given the antispasmodic drug Bentyl to take when I felt an attack was imminent.

> "This should really help with the pain that you are feeling during these attacks. It helps to calm the muscles in the GI tract and prevent them from going into spasm."

Was this medicine going to work? Isn't this an antispasmodic just like Levsin that Dr. Hamilton gave to me? I had hope that possibly this would do the trick. I so desperately wanted to be able to go out in public and not worry about having an attack.

> *Bentyl, also known as dicyclomine, is an anticholinergic drug used in the treatment of irritable bowel syndrome (IBS). It causes the smooth muscle in the gastrointestinal tract to relax by blocking a chemical present in the intestines.*

Around this time, my husband and I took at trip to Milwaukee to visit my family. I had my Bentyl on hand, so I wasn't as panicked about having an attack during the trip. I figured if an attack started up, I would immediately take the Bentyl. I wouldn't wait for a full blown attack. Our first day there was very enjoyable, and at the end of the day we all sat around the television and watched a movie.

As the movie was ending, I suddenly started to feel weird and my stomach started to bloat. It was around 11 p.m., so I told everyone that I was going to get ready for bed. As I was doing so, I really started to feel sick, so I took a Bentyl. Then the cramps hit! I spent the next 30 minutes or so in the bathroom patiently waiting for the Bentyl to kick in while I was sweating and doubled over from the severe pain. Much to my dismay, the Bentyl never relieved any of the pain. In fact, this turned out to be one of the worst attacks that I had ever had. I was vomiting, had diarrhea, and my stomach was so bloated that I looked pregnant again. The rest of the trip was not too enjoyable to me as I was afraid to eat anything and was scared to go anywhere for fear of another attack. To this day, I am shocked that I was even able to get back on the plane to get home.

After this trip, I had to leave my job. In addition to the debilitating pain, the depression and stress became so severe that I was unable to work. I felt like the life I knew was coming to an end, and I didn't know why.

I didn't go back to the doctor after this. I was convinced at this point that no one could help me. No doctor in that little town knew what was going on with me. It was then that I realized the only person who would be able to help me was me, so I decided to do my own research. I quickly realized that my diet needed some changing. As you will see in the next chapter, the changes that I made in my diet at this time did actually help to reduce some of my symptoms.

Improvement with Diet

At this point in my life, I was feeling alone, desperate and very depressed. I did not know where to turn for help. I finally realized that if I wanted to see any change in this pattern of pain, I needed to help myself by doing my own research.

I started to read about nutrition. I had never really thought too much about what I ate during the day. I just ate what I wanted to eat. As I was educating myself on nutrition, I came to realize how poor my food choices had been over the years. I was eating a lot of processed food and very little fresh food. My fruit and vegetable intake was quite low, and I ate a lot of fast food since I was always "on the go". Additionally, my husband and I always looked for food that was "no fat", thinking at the time that this was the healthy way to eat. We couldn't have been more wrong!

One day, my husband read an article in Prevention magazine about the health benefits of omega-3 fatty acids. This was a real eye-opener for us. We couldn't believe the benefits that this little fatty acid has on the human body. So, we ordered a large container of ground flaxseed meal and started to sprinkle it on certain foods - oatmeal, spaghetti sauce, etc. It doesn't have much of a taste to it, so we couldn't even tell we were eating it when we added it to our food. Around the same time, I started to eat more fruits and vegetables. Within several months, I saw a dramatic reduction in the severity of my attacks of abdominal pain. I was shocked but so happy! The attacks didn't disappear, but they weren't nearly as severe.

I continued to do more research and dramatically changed my diet. At work I began eating salads containing lettuce, shredded cheese, olives, broccoli, cauliflower, green peppers, banana peppers, cucumbers, red onions and tomatoes. I would eat this for lunch for 4 to 5 days out of the week. We continued to sprinkle flaxseed meal on our food at home, and we started taking a daily fish oil supplement. I also took a daily multivitamin.

I changed my breakfast food from a bagel and cream cheese to a bowl of oatmeal. I routinely made baked salmon as I was trying to eat fish at least once a week. I stopped buying white bread and instead started buying multigrain or wheat bread for sandwiches. I discovered edamame and crab around this time and these foods quickly became two of my favorites. I began to use olive oil in most of my recipes. I began to cook more and found out how tasty food became when using fresh garlic. To this day, I will end up using about an entire garlic bulb in my recipes per week! Since I learned that lemon can help to detoxify the liver, I started to add fresh lemon juice to my glasses of water. I have recently found a delicious way to prepare tuna fish, and I also have a great homemade hummus recipe that includes lots of garlic and olive oil. These have also become some of my favorites.

Since I saw such a dramatic decrease in my symptoms, I began to work toward a Master's degree in Holistic Nutrition from Clayton College of Natural Health. I decided to do some further research into omega-3 fatty acids and irritable bowel syndrome which led to my thesis, "The Effects of Omega-3 Fatty Acids on Irritable Bowel Syndrome and Inflammatory Bowel Disease". I was so passionate about this thesis since it involved my own personal experience, and I'm proud to say that the first draft was approved by the college.

At this point, I was convinced that I did have irritable bowel syndrome and that my change in diet would finally fix the problem. But not so fast....the story continues.....

34

The Later Years

In November 1997, my husband and I moved to the Washington, DC area. Although the attacks of severe abdominal pain were better, I still was having milder versions of the attacks. My stomach was still bloating up severely at the end of my period, and I was still having dysfunctional uterine bleeding. Since my husband and I wanted children, I discontinued the birth control pill so we could try to conceive. However, after several years of trying, I was never able to become pregnant. So, although diet clearly helped me, I believed the root cause of the problem still had not been addressed. When we arrived in the DC area, I did my research and found a highly ranked family practice doctor. In November, 1998, I had my first appointment with Dr. Mattington.

I explained to Dr. Mattington that I had a history of left sided abdominal pain associated with my period with sweating, shakiness, and a fast heart rate. I was 33 years old during this first visit with her. After discussing my medical history at length with her, she too was at a loss for what was actually happening to me. According to her report,

> *"Unclear to me what is happening - episodic but regular attacks, clearly related to the menstrual cycle. Raised possibility of panic attacks perhaps triggered by hormone surges. Plan gynecological evaluation."*

Dr. Mattington referred me to a highly ranked gynecologist in the area. She also did a complete blood workup to rule out any other problem that might be contributing to these attacks. The tests performed included a comprehensive metabolic panel, urinary catecholamines and urine VMA. All of these tests came back normal. Additionally, she started me on Ortho Novum 777 - another birth control pill - since I was starting to bleed heavily again. I was hesitant about doing this since my husband and I were trying to have children, but the quality of my life was really suffering.

I scheduled an appointment with the gynecologist, Dr. Seale. However, she was in such high demand that I had to wait for two months before I could get an appointment. Although frustrated at the thought of having to wait, I agreed to set up an appointment with her in January, 1999.

About a week later, I was driving on the interstate on the way to work when out of the blue, my stomach started to bloat again. I started to get dizzy and shaky, and then my heart started to race. I was worried I wouldn't be able to make it to work. I also had mild nausea and what felt like heartburn. I tried to slow down my breathing and relax as I was in the middle of traffic and by myself. I did make it to work, and everything seemed to settle down once I was there. That day, I went back to Dr. Mattington and told her what had happened that morning on the interstate. At the time, she thought I might have had heartburn and she gave me a prescription for Prilosec, but looking back on it now, I think I was having a panic attack.

Prilosec, also known as omeprazole, in a proton pump inhibitor that is used to decrease acid production in the stomach. It is used in the treatment of gastroesophageal reflux disease (GERD).

In January, 1999, I had my first appointment with the gynecologist, Dr. Seale. I had a great deal of hope going into this appointment because she was in high demand which made me think she had to be a good doctor. When I first saw her, I was taking Ortho Novum 777 for management of the abnormal bleeding and severe abdominal pain, and I was taking Levsin as needed for management of pain from IBS. During the pelvic exam, she noted that the uterus was "anteverted". This is basically considered a normal variant and is not thought to pose any problems, so it was noted but not addressed any further.

There are several known positions of the uterus which can occur as a normal variant or be a result of adhesions from endometriosis as this may "pull" the uterus in certain directions. Also, pain from fibroid tumors in the uterus will be felt in different areas according to the position of the uterus. In an anteversion, the uterus is tilted toward the front of the abdomen. Pain from fibroids in this case is more likely felt in the front of the abdomen. Conversely, in retroversion, the uterus is tilted more toward the back, and so pain from fibroids is more likely to be felt in the patient's back.

According to her report, her impressions and plan were as follows:

1. *Pelvic pain episodes*
2. *History of endometriosis*
3. *Spastic colon*
4. *Delayed conception*

"Begin taking 800 mg Motrin on first day of menses as an anti-prostaglandin preventative. Refer for consult regarding in vitro fertilization. Perform day 3 labs."

I went to the lab on day 3 of my menstrual cycle and had several tubes of blood drawn. The following tests were performed:

Follicle stimulating hormone (FSH)
Luteinizing hormone (LH)
Prolactin
DHEA sulfate
Estradiol
Amenorrhea profile
Thyroid stimulating hormone (TSH)

Every one of these tests came back in the normal range. This was noted and placed in my chart, and we continued with Motrin and Ortho Novum 777 to try and control the pain and dysfunctional bleeding.

My next appointment was a consultation regarding in vitro fertilization and a discussion on my inability to get pregnant. Since all previous testing had shown no abnormalities other than a very small amount of endometriosis, we decided to stop the Ortho Novum 777. After several months, I was started on Clomid to increase the number of eggs released every month. After six months of treatment, I still was unable to become pregnant so I decided to stop this hormone as it was causing me some unwanted side effects such as nausea and hot flashes. My husband and I decided to let nature take its course. We prayed a lot and decided to leave it in God's hands. If He wanted us to have children, somehow we would.

Clomid, also known as Clomiphene, induces ovulation by binding to estrogen receptors. This tricks the body into thinking estrogen levels are low. As a result, there is a surge in the levels of FSH and LH. This triggers ovulation. This drug is used to treat female infertility. The following are possible symptoms with the use of Clomid:

Nausea
Vomiting
Diarrhea
Flushing (hot flashes)
Breast tenderness
Abnormal vaginal bleeding
Headache
Fatigue
Vaginal dryness
Blurred vision
Depression

Use of this drug can lead to multiple births. Additionally, Clomid is listed as a pregnancy category X drug, meaning that this drug is known to cause birth defects. Contraindications for use of Clomid include:

Undiagnosed vaginal bleeding
Endometriosis
Uterine fibroids

I had another follow up with Dr. Seale in June, 1999. We discussed our decision about having children, and the exam proved once again to be normal. I continued on the road of a healthy diet, Motrin and Ortho Novum 777.

In March, 2000, a friend of mine told me about a condition called celiac sprue. Since I had been suffering for so long with the gastrointestinal issues, she suggested that I might want to be tested for this condition. I made an appointment with Dr. Mattington and discussed this with her. Celiac sprue is a digestive disorder where the intestine is unable to process a substance in foods called gluten. Could this have been the problem all along? I strongly considered this because I saw such a dramatic decrease in my symptoms when I changed my diet. I had reduced my consumption of bread which contains a high amount of gluten. Maybe this was the problem! My doctor agreed to have me tested for this condition; however, when the results came back, they were negative. Again, it was a bittersweet moment. I didn't have celiac sprue so I could continue to eat anything I wanted, but I still didn't have an answer to the cause of this abdominal pain.

The yeast infections were continuing. I kept wondering if other women were having as much of an issue with yeast infections. I knew that birth control pills could increase the risk of yeast infections, but this seemed excessive to me. I was starting to get really sick of buying Monistat!

Then one night in December of 2000, I had one of the worst attacks of abdominal pain that I had ever had up to this point. I woke up in the middle of the night with extremely severe cramping on my left side that would move down into my pelvic area. This lasted for several hours followed by two hours of constant diarrhea. During the cramping, there were several times when I thought for sure that I was going to faint. During the height of the cramp, I would get so dizzy that I would start to see stars. All I could do was wait it out and pray to God,

"Please don't let me pass out, please don't let me pass out. Please get me through this, God!"

The next day, I was off to see Dr. Mattington once again. When she came into the room, I was in tears. I just couldn't take it anymore. She was so sympathetic and understanding, but her response was the same:

"I'm so sorry, but I'm still not sure what's going on here."

I could see the sympathy in her eyes, and I know she did care. I'm sure she was just as frustrated about this as I was.

I was once again diagnosed with IBS. She gave me another prescription for Bentyl, but I had no hope that this was going to help since it didn't do anything for me the first time it was prescribed. Since I had what felt like terrible constipation during the first half of the attack before I started to have diarrhea, she recommended that I drink prune juice and take magnesium citrate to help to regulate the function of my intestinal tract. I agreed and left the office frustrated more than ever.

Around this same time, I started to notice that my menstrual periods were becoming heavier, longer and more painful. In addition, I was passing very large blood clots during my period, sometimes as big as the palm of my hand, and I was having terrible migraine headaches. I also noticed that I was feeling a great deal of pressure on my bladder during my period and was constantly having to run to the bathroom. I went for in for another appointment with Dr. Seale.

I felt at this point that Dr. Seale was getting frustrated with me. I kept coming back to her with the same complaints over and over again, but she couldn't find a concrete reason why I was having so much trouble. She didn't seem to want to spend the time with me, and I felt very rushed to get through the appointment. This only added to my already high stress level regarding my severe abdominal pain and other menstrual issues.

I left the office with the diagnosis of menstrual migraines and a prescription for Imitrex. I was told to watch and see if I continued to pass blood clots with my periods. If it continued over the next several months, she told me that I might need to have an endometrial biopsy.

Imitrex, also known as sumatriptan, is in the class of selective serotonin receptor agonist class of drugs. It is used in the treatment of migraine headaches by narrowing the blood vessels in the brain. Side effects include drowsiness, dizziness, nausea, vomiting, diarrhea, flushing, tingling, and muscle cramps.

After this appointment, I went quite a long time before going back because I was so frustrated and irritated with doctors in general. I was convinced that no one was going to be able to help me. I would have to put up with this for the rest of my life! In February 2001, I had my annual physical with Dr. Mattington. I explained to her that my abdominal pain issues were continuing along with my menstrual problems, and because of this, I was having a hard time with depression. She decided to prescribe Sarafem for me to help with the depression and possible pre-menstrual dysphoric disorder (PMDD).

Sarafem, also known as fluoxetine or Prozac, is a well-known antidepressant medication. It has also been used to treat premenstrual dysphoric disorder, obsessive-compulsive disorder, and panic attacks. It works by increasing serotonin levels in the brain, and it is in the class of selective serotonin re-uptake inhibitor drugs (SSRIs).

Premenstrual dysphoric disorder refers to a severe form of PMS. Symptoms typically start a week before a menstrual period and continue until a few days after a period starts. The depression, tension and anxiety are worse than typical PMS. It affects 3 to 8% of all women, and hormone changes play a major role. Symptoms include the following:

Fatigue
Severe anxiety
Severe sadness or hopelessness
Being "on edge"
Marked anger
Food cravings
Binge eating
Bloating
Breast tenderness
Headaches
Muscle pain
Insomnia
Severe mood swings
Concentration problems
Suicidal thoughts

These symptoms can be severe and disabling.

During that same month, I had my annual pap and pelvic exam. This time, I decided to write down on paper all of my pre-menstrual symptoms so that my gynecologist would have all of the information about my condition. The following is the list that I gave to her:

About 4-5 days before period -

1. Severe moodiness - uncontrollable crying
2. Extremely bad depression - feeling out of control, can't deal with stress, feeling overwhelmed.
3. Severe breast pain in left breast only. Normal exam and mammogram except for fibrocystic disease.
4. Insomnia - some nights only getting 2 to 3 hours of sleep.
5. Horrible headaches - possible migraines, have Imitrex.
6. Heartbeat problems - feeling like it skips a beat and getting dizzy/lightheaded.

7. Extreme appetite fluctuations - sometimes there is near constant hunger, other times no appetite and nausea.
8. Extreme fatigue - unable to concentrate
9. Excessive urination
10. Shakiness

Fibrocystic breast disease refers to painful, swollen and lumpy breasts. This disorder affects over 50 percent of women and does not increase a woman's risk for breast cancer.

Although I brought this list in to her, she just tossed it to the side and did the annual exam. She didn't find any abnormalities during the exam, so I guess she just thought this was all in my head.

Several months later, I had a particularly bad menstrual cycle. Symptoms included severe cramping, hot flashes, night sweats, vomiting, and passing blood clots. I returned once again to Dr. Seale. This time during the exam, she said that there was a possibility that I had a tiny fibroid present in the uterus. I was told to stop the birth control pill and start on Ponstel. We would observe what effect this was having on my menstrual cycle for 2-3 months and then decide if a laparoscopy or other procedure would be necessary. So, I filled the prescription and began to take Ponstel.

Ponstel, also known as mefenamic acid, is in a class of drugs called NSAIDS. It is used to treat mild to moderate pain and is most frequently used to treat menstrual cramps. Side effects include bloating, constipation, diarrhea, dizziness nervousness, heartburn, nausea and ringing in the ears. This drug puts the patient at an increased risk for heart attack and stroke.

A fibroid tumor, also known as a leiomyoma is a mass found in the uterine wall. It is a benign tumor, and estrogen has been shown to stimulate its growth. Symptoms include heavy bleeding that can lead to anemia, pelvic pain, pressure on the bladder, and painful bowel movements. In addition, fibroids may interfere with fertility.

The Ponstel was ineffective. I continued with the abdominal pain and blood clots during my period. I was also having PMDD, chills, nausea, and hot flashes. During my follow up visit with the gynecologist, she decided to discontinue the Ponstel and try a continuous dose of Yasmin instead. This continuous birth control treatment would mean that I would have a menstrual period only 4 times per year. In addition, she increased my dose of Sarafem. So for the umpteenth time I was sent home with different medication in hopes that this time I would get some relief.

Yasmin is a birth control pill that contains drospirenone (progesterone) and ethinyl estradiol (estrogen). Studies have shown that drospirenone in this birth control pill is linked to an increase in the incidence of blood clots. Additionally, Yasmin may increase potassium levels in the body.

Several weeks after starting on Yasmin, I started to develop a crampy feeling in my right leg. It felt like my calf muscle was constantly cramping. All during the day at work, I would flex my right foot up to try and get it to stop cramping. After about a week of this, I started to do some research. I found out that this symptom might actually be a sign of deep vein thrombosis (DVT) in someone who is taking Yasmin. So, I went back to see my gynecologist.

Dr. Seale came into the room, quickly looked at my leg, and determined that this was not DVT. She told me that she wasn't too concerned since my leg wasn't red or swollen. However, years later I learned that DVT was a major issue with women who had been on Yasmin. In fact, lawsuits have been filed against the manufacturer regarding blood clots with this pill. Of note is the fact that this cramping pain in my right leg stopped once I stopped taking Yasmin. Was this in fact a developing blood clot in my right leg? We'll never know for sure.

Finally, in April, 2002, I had enough. This time, during yet another follow up visit with my gynecologist, I was adamant about doing further testing to see what was going on with me. She agreed to send me to have a transabdominal and transvaginal ultrasound to get a good look at what was going on inside my uterus. According to the radiologist report, the uterus was levoverted. This means that it was leaning over toward the left side of my abdomen. Additionally, the radiologist stated the following:

"Endometrial lining: 5 mm in thickness but there is evidence for a possible 5 mm polyp along the LEFT side of the fundal endometrium. Consider hysteroscopy or sonohysterography."

45

An endometrial or uterine polyp is a growth protruding from the uterine wall into the uterus. It is usually benign, but there have been cases where they become cancerous. It comes from overgrowth of the endometrium and it is estrogen sensitive. Symptoms include infertility, irregular or heavy periods, and bleeding between periods.

A sonohysterogram was scheduled to be performed the following month to get a better image of this polyp that had been found in the upper part of my uterus.

A sonohysterogram is a minimally invasive procedure that is used to visualize and evaluate uterine abnormalities such as fibroids and polyps. This procedure is also used to evaluate women who suffer from infertility or repeated miscarriages. A transvaginal ultrasound is done first to locate abnormalities and examine the inside of the uterus. When this is done, the probe is removed and a speculum is inserted. The cervix is cleansed, and a small catheter is placed into the uterus. Next, the speculum is removed and the transvaginal ultrasound probe is reinserted. Sterile saline is injected into the uterus through the catheter, and the ultrasound is performed. The entire procedure usually takes about 30 minutes to perform. Most women tolerate the procedure well, although there may be some cramping.

About a month later, I went in for my sonohysterogram. A friend of mine had an endometrial biopsy several years before, and she had told me about how painful it was for her to have this test done. Although this was not the exact same test, I knew that they would be entering into my uterus with a small tube, so I expected this to be somewhat painful. So, needless to say, I was a nervous wreck!

A transvaginal ultrasound was done prior to the sonohysterogram. This test had been performed on me before, so I wasn't too nervous about that portion of the exam. After the ultrasound was done, a small tube was threaded up through my cervix and into the uterus. I was pleasantly surprised when I didn't feel any pain. Then the doctor told me that they were going to inject some fluid into the uterine cavity so that they could visualize the polyp a little better. He said that I might have some cramping pain during this part of the test, but again I was surprised when I didn't feel any pain. He took pictures of the polyp, and I watched on the ultrasound screen as all of this was happening. When it was over, I was so happy. This wasn't nearly as bad as I had expected. But I spoke too fast.

As my husband and I were driving home after the test, my stomach suddenly started to bloat. I looked like I was pregnant again. That horrible abdominal pain hit me as we were stuck in the middle of a traffic jam. Here I was, doubled over in pain, feeling sick and faint, and we couldn't move at all. I just sat there, breathing deep while trying to get through the pain, and praying that I didn't vomit in the car. Finally, the traffic started to move, and my husband was able to stop at a Wendy's restaurant so I could use the bathroom. Luckily, after having a bowel movement, the pain quickly resolved and my stomach returned to its normal size. At this point, I just knew in my heart that this abdominal pain was in some way definitely linked to my uterus. What are the chances that a severe attack of IBS would happen right after having an invasive procedure involving my uterus? I really started to believe that my gastrointestinal tract wasn't the problem - it was the uterus. Now, getting my doctors to agree with this would be another story.

The following is an excerpt from the radiologist's report regarding my sonohysterogram:

"The preliminary transabdominal study shows the uterus to be normal for size measuring 7.4 cm for length. No adnexal abnormality is seen. No free fluid in the pelvis. Following prepping of the cervix, a 5 French catheter was introduced through the cervical os and a small amount of sterile saline was injected during ultrasound observation. A broad based pedunculated endometrial polyp is seen at the level of the uterine midbody just to the LEFT of midline with a maximum diameter of 7 mm. The polyp is estimated to be approximately 4 cm from the level of the cervix. The endometrium is otherwise thin and uniform with single wall thickness of 1-2 mm."

At some point during this time, I was switched to yet another birth control pill. This time, my doctor wanted me to try continuous Lo-Estrin. I stayed on this pill for the next several years.

The next step was to schedule a hysteroscopy for removal of the endometrial polyp. This surgery was scheduled for October, 2002. During this surgery, it was noted that I had cervical stenosis and a septate bicornuate uterus.

Cervical stenosis refers to the opening of the cervix being smaller than what is normally seen.

After so many years of being seen by so many doctors, this is the first time that I had heard that I had a bicornuate uterus.

A bicornuate uterus is also known as a "heart-shaped" uterus. This type of uterus has two "horns" which occurs as a result of a congenital abnormality of the fusion of the Mullerian ducts during fetal development. It occurs in 0.1 to 0.5% of women, and pregnancies in these women are considered high risk. Problems during pregnancy in someone with a bicornuate uterus include:

> *Cervical incompetence*
> *Repeat pregnancy loss (miscarriage)*
> *Pre-term births*
> *Breech births*
> *Retained placenta*
> *Birth defects*

The following is an excerpt from the operative report from my hysteroscopy:

"The cervix was grasped with a tooth tenaculum and an attempt was made to sound the uterus. The uterine sound was unable to be passed through the cervix. A tonsil hemostat was then used to attempt to dilate the cervix. This was unsuccessful. Then, an os finder was used to successfully dilate the cervix. The uterus sounded to 8 cm. Using Pratt graduated dilators the cervix was dilated sufficiently to admit the 0 degree hysteroscope. The hysteroscope was inserted using glycine as the distention medium. The endocervix appeared normal. Just inside the level of the internal os there was a polyp noted that had a smooth, pale surface. It was linear and may have even represented a small fibroid. Thy hysteroscope was advanced further and it was noted that the uterus had a slightly septate bicornuate appearance. The right horn was rather shallow. The left

horn was deeper. The endometrium itself appeared pale and unremarkable. The right ostia was visualized. The left ostium was difficult to visualize; however, the left horn appeared somewhat narrow and was difficult to be certain whether the ostium was identified. The hysteroscope was removed. The Corson polyp forceps were introduced yielding a 1 cm x 7mm, firm, polypoid mass consistent with either polyp or small fibroids. The small uterine curet was then used to curet the endometrial surface yielding moderate tissue. The hysteroscope was then reintroduced showing the resolution of the polypoid mass and freshly curetted endometrium."

The pathology report from this surgery stated the following:

"Endometrial polyp, fragments of endometrium showing atrophic glands with mild decidual change of stroma consistent with hormone effect."

After the surgery, there were no complications. I recovered for a few days at home and then resumed my normal activities.

During my post op visit, Dr. Seale explained that the dysfunctional uterine bleeding that I had been experiencing was probably a result of the polyp that was present in my uterus. She believed that removal of this polyp would resolve a lot of the symptoms that I had been experiencing. This would be my last visit with her because my husband was transferred to Texas, and we were in the process of a major move.

I left the Washington, DC area on a continuous birth control pill (LoEstrin) and I would only have 4 menstrual periods per year. I was still taking Sarafem for depression, and I had just had an endometrial polyp removed from my uterus. Everything was under control, but I still believed that the root cause of my issues had not been determined.

Hysterectomy and Discovery of Adenomyosis

My husband and I moved to San Antonio, Texas in the summer of 2003. The doctors in the Washington, DC area had controlled my symptoms by putting me on a continuous birth control pill where I would only have a period 4 times per year. I was on an antidepressant, Sarafem, and I had recently had an endometrial polyp removed from my uterus through a hysteroscopy. During this surgery, I learned that I had a bicornuate uterus that was also levoverted. Although the symptoms had been managed, I still knew in my heart that the root cause of all these years of pain and suffering had not yet been discovered. I was basically treating the symptoms, but the main problem was still there.

My symptoms seemed to remain under control for several years. I didn't want to change what had been prescribed for fear that all of the problems would return full force, so I just stayed with the program as it was when I left Washington. However, things started to go downhill in 2006. I started to have some bad attacks of abdominal pain with severe stomach bloating that would just hit me out of the blue. One morning I was getting ready to leave for work, and all of a sudden my stomach bloated up to the size of about a 4 month pregnancy. A few minutes later I was doubled over in pain and actually had to crawl to the bathroom. In the middle of this, I somehow managed to crawl to the phone and called in to work saying that I would be there when the attack let up.

The continuous birth control therapy helped me because I was only having four periods a year. However, when the periods did come, they were increasingly long, sometimes lasting a full two weeks. The bleeding was extremely heavy, and I would have terrible cramping along with bad PMS. The fatigue and headaches were debilitating, and there were many days I would come home from work and go straight to bed without even eating dinner. I was passing very large blood clots and was also dizzy and lightheaded, probably due to the amount of blood I was shedding. I finally had enough. I did my research and found a new highly ranked gynecologist in Texas. This time I hit the jackpot!

But relief didn't come immediately. I was very impressed when I first met Dr. Kramer. Of all the doctors that I had seen over the years, this one seemed the most concerned. She did my exam and noticed no abnormalities, confirming what my previous doctors had told me. However, she was still very worried. Since I was in my 40's by this time, and my husband and I had accepted the fact that I wasn't going to get pregnant, she discussed the option of having an endometrial ablation.

An endometrial ablation is a medical procedure that destroys the endometrium inside the uterus. This procedure is typically done on women who are suffering from excessive blood loss during menstruation and in cases where medication is ineffective to control this blood loss. The procedure can be done many different ways, from using extreme cold, heated liquids, microwave energy, radiofrequency or through electrosurgery. This procedure is not recommended for patients in the following circumstances:

Those who wish to become pregnant in the future
Those who have known uterine cancer
Those who have recently had a baby
Those who are post menopausal

For those women who still wish to have children, endometrial ablation is not a viable option because this procedure damages the lining of the uterus. Although periods usually stop after having this procedure, there have still been reports of pregnancy occurring after an endometrial ablation. These pregnancies usually end in miscarriage.

An incision is not necessary during this procedure. The tools required for an ablation are inserted into the uterus through the cervix. Depending on the method chosen the endometrium is destroyed, the tools are removed, and the patient is allowed to recover for several hours. After the procedure, the patient may feel cramping pain and have a watery or bloody discharge for a few weeks. The results of this procedure are either lighter periods or cessation of menstruation. It is imperative to continue to use some form of contraception as the risk of miscarriage is quite high after an ablation.

After discussing this at length with my husband, we decided to go ahead with the surgery and started the preparing for the big day.

On the day of the surgery, I was a little nervous, but I had endured so many procedures and surgeries that it really didn't bother me much anymore. I just wanted to get it over with so I could go on with my life without any more pain and bleeding problems. I was actually happy when the nurses came to take me into surgery.

I came out of surgery without any complications. I recovered for several hours and was released to go home later that day. The next two days at home were uneventful with no pain or bleeding. I really thought that the problems of the past seventeen years had finally come to an end. But, I was wrong....

On the third day after surgery, I woke up to find that I was bleeding fairly heavily. This clearly should not have been happening. I waited for a day to see if it would resolve itself, but it didn't. My husband drove me to the hospital the next morning where I explained to them that I had just had an endometrial ablation. The ER doctor performed a pelvic exam on me which for some reason was extraordinarily painful. She noted the bleeding but couldn't give me a reason to why it was happening. She suggested that I return to Dr. Kramer for further treatment.

The next day, we went to see Dr. Kramer. She performed a pelvic exam and stated that this is the first time she had seen this much blood loss after an endometrial ablation. She told me that this was clearly abnormal and was very concerned about my condition. It was at this point that I asked her to perform a hysterectomy. She agreed, and we moved forward to schedule the surgery.

Several weeks later, I was at the hospital getting ready to have a hysterectomy. We had agreed that removal of the uterus was all that was necessary at the time. The hysterectomy was going to be a laparoscopic procedure. Dr. Kramer explained to me that with this kind of procedure, there is a possibility that she would not be able to get all of the uterine tissue removed during surgery. This meant that I may continue to have light spotting during the time of menstruation after the surgery and until menopause. She was also going to leave the ovaries in place to prevent premature menopause. I was so relieved to be at this place in my life. I felt deep in my heart that the uterus was the problem all along, and finally a doctor has agreed to take it out. I thought that maybe this time I will finally get some relief and some peace!

The surgery went very well. I did not have any complications. My mom came to Texas to be with me during this time, and her support was a tremendous comfort to me. I was up and walking around the day after surgery, and she couldn't believe that I came out of it as easily as I did. The morning after surgery, I had one small bout of abdominal pain that lasted about 15 minutes, but it resolved rather quickly after I had a bowel movement. A few days later, we had a post op appointment with Dr. Kramer. Little did I know, but this appointment would give me the answers that I had been looking for for the past seventeen years.

My mom and I sat patiently in the room as we waited for Dr. Kramer to come in to see me. She finally came in, sat down and looked at me.

"Well, I have the pathology results from your hysterectomy. It turns out that you had a condition called adenomyosis. There were also multiple small fibroid tumors found throughout the uterine wall."

She proceeded to tell me all about this disorder. Everything she said to me sounded exactly like what I had experienced over the past 17 years. This was it - this is the day that I had been waiting for! It was finally over!

The next day, I sent roses to Dr. Kramer. I wanted her to know how much it meant to me that she was finally able to properly diagnose my condition and give me the peace that I had been searching for all of those years.

Since my hysterectomy, I have never had a recurrence of an attack of severe abdominal pain. It has been six years, and all of my symptoms are gone since the removal of my uterus. In the end, this pain had nothing at all to do with IBS. All of the procedures and medications used for the treatment of IBS were worthless in my case. This was entirely a problem with the uterus.....a little known condition called adenomyosis. The next chapter gives all the information currently known about this disorder.

Although I finally got relief from the abdominal pain that had been causing all this suffering for 17 years, other health problems continued to bother me and even new things started to happen.

My allergy situation, which had been under control for years, started to return. I had finished the allergy shots, and I was slowly starting to have more and more sinus trouble with each passing year. Then, I started to notice a weird pattern. I would have a flare up of sinus congestion each month during my PMS time. My head would be so congested during this time, and I was constantly blowing my nose and having sinus headaches. Once the menstrual spotting would start, my sinus congestion would clear up until the next month. I thought this was strange, and I just could not imagine at all that sinus congestion could somehow be linked to female hormone fluctuations. I could not have been more surprised when I did my research and found out that this symptom could be linked to estrogen dominance which will be discussed later in this book.

Just as I was getting used to feeling good, yet another health issue hit me out of the blue. In the spring of 2009 as I was getting out of bed one morning, my right leg suddenly gave out from underneath me. I found out that I had a herniated disc in my lumbar back and I needed to have a spinal fusion. In September of that same year, I had the fusion and was told after the surgery that one of the vertebrae in my lower back was actually broken. I had hoped that this surgery would fix the problem, but it didn't. The bones failed to fuse, so I had a second surgery in 2010. Interestingly enough, the second surgery also failed. For some reason that could not be identified, the bones in my lower spine were failing to fuse. I did not have any risk factors for fusion failure, so this was puzzling not only to me but also to my doctors. I had a third spinal fusion in 2012. This time, in addition to using the routine hardware (rods and screws), bone morphogenic protein and bone marrow that was aspirated from my hip were used to aid in fusion. I had been found to be low in vitamin D, so I was put on a prescription vitamin D pill during this time. Thankfully, with all the extra effort put into the third surgery, it did succeed and the bones finally fused.

Little did I know at the time that these fusion failures might have been caused by the same thing as my adenomyosis!

All About Adenomyosis

Adenomyosis is a uterine disorder. This condition has also been referred to as "endometriosis interna" and is characterized by the presence of endometrial tissue inside the myometrial layer of the uterus. Although this condition is sometimes associated with endometriosis, in reality the two diseases are completely separate problems, and both disorders are found together in just ten percent of cases. Sound confusing? Here's a quick lesson on the anatomy of the uterus, and hopefully this will help you to understand adenomyosis a little better.

The uterus basically has two layers, the endometrium and the myometrium. The inner layer is the endometrium, and this layer thickens each month through the effects of hormones. This layer is shed each month in the form of a menstrual period. The outer layer is the muscular layer and is called the myometrium. This muscular layer contracts each month to help the body rid itself of the endometrium which causes the pain that is felt with menstrual cramps. Additionally the myometrium is the muscle that contracts during childbirth. In a normal uterus, the endometrium and the myometrium are two distinct layers and do not invade each other.

However, in adenomyosis, the endometrium for unknown reasons invades and works its way into the myometrium. When a woman's menstrual cycle occurs in someone with adenomyosis, the cramping pain is severe due to the fact that blood (endometrial tissue) is trapped inside the uterine muscle. This condition is usually found in women between the ages of 35 and 50. It can be spread sporadically throughout the uterine muscle, or it can cause a larger growth in one area called an adenomyoma.

Why does the endometrium end up inside the myometrium? We don't know. There are several theories, but the bottom line is that no one is certain of the cause. At one point, some doctors thought that retrograde menstruation or a "backward flow" might be the cause. However, this currently is viewed as a very unlikely cause of either adenomyosis or endometriosis. More current thinking is that any procedure where the barrier between the endometrium and myometrium has been compromised might lead to the condition. Examples of this include pregnancy, pregnancy termination, D&C, caesarean section, etc. It has also been proposed that since this disorder usually shows up between the ages of 35 and 50, estrogen dominance may play a role as this is usually the time in a woman's life when progesterone levels decrease and there may be an excess of estrogen present in the body. Other studies suggest that other hormones may play a role

61

including follicle stimulating hormone and prolactin. It is clear that its growth is dependent on circulating estrogen in the body. At menopause, production of estrogen decreases and symptoms of adenomyosis diminish.

Estrogen dominance is of particular interest here. When this happens, estrogen outweighs the level of progesterone in the body. Basically this is just a hormonal imbalance. Most often, this condition is a result of low progesterone levels with normal levels of estrogen. Just because an estrogen level appears to be normal does not mean that estrogen dominance is not at play. If the progesterone level is low and the estrogen level is normal, that means that unopposed estrogen is present in the body, and that person is affected by estrogen dominance. This condition is also exacerbated by stress. Additionally, this condition is not generally recognized in western medicine. It is usually noted by naturopathic physicians.

A physician may or may not be able to pick up adenomyosis when doing a pelvic exam. The uterus may be soft, tender and slightly enlarged. A mass may be felt if an adenomyoma is present. Also, the uterus becomes heavier with more diffuse involvement of adenomyosis. During surgery, the uterus may appear normal or abnormal, depending on the degree of involvement of the adenomyosis. If the adenomyosis is encased entirely within the uterine muscle, it will not be able to be visualized during surgery, and the uterus will appear normal. Adenomyosis is often misdiagnosed as fibroids (leiomyomas).

At the current time, the only way to get a definitive diagnosis of adenomyosis is during a hysterectomy. This disorder can usually only be detected from looking at uterine tissue underneath a microscope, and this is typically performed by a pathologist. A hysterectomy is usually necessary to get a definitive diagnosis. The disorder usually can only be detected by looking at all of the uterine tissue since adenomyosis is usually seen in sporadic areas of the uterine muscle. To control the symptoms of adenomyosis, the uterus needs to be removed. The ovaries can remain intact. A biopsy of the uterine wall without hysterectomy may or may not detect the disorder depending if the biopsy site contains the adenomyosis. If this disorder is strongly suspected but hysterectomy is not an option, multiple biopsies of the uterine wall can be taken, but luck would play a big factor in whether or not these biopsy sites contained the adenomyosis. At the current time, hysterectomy and examination of the entire uterus after its removal is the only way to get a definitive diagnosis of adenomyosis. MRI is showing a little hope in picking up large adenomyomas without the need for hysterectomy, but this test generally will not pick up small scattered areas of adenomyosis in the uterine wall.

The symptoms of adenomyosis include the following:

Painful menstrual bleeding (dysmennorhea)
Heavy menstrual bleeding (menorrhagia)
Severe abdominal cramping (sometimes can be as severe as the last stage of labor)
Enlarged, bulky and heavy uterus (often doubling or tripling in size)
Tenderness during pelvic exam
Severe bloating
A "bearing down" sensation
Heaviness in the legs
Bleeding between periods
Painful intercourse
Pressure on the bladder
Painful bowel movements during menstruation
Passing large blood clots
Prolonged menstrual bleeding (8 to 14 days)
Chronic anemia
Depression, anxiety
May contribute to infertility
Increase in pain over time - can be debilitating
More common as women age
Some women have no symptoms

So how is it treated if it is found prior to a hysterectomy? Usually, treatment is only effective if the adenomyosis is limited to one particular area in the uterine muscle, as can be seen in an adenomyoma. In these cases, the adenomyoma can be cauterized or excised and can provide good symptom relief. However, in most cases, the adenomyosis is scattered throughout the uterine muscle and is not limited to one area. This is very hard to treat without doing a hysterectomy. Endometrial ablations have been tried in these cases but are typically unsuccessful. This is because an ablation only affects the surface layer of the endometrium. The adenomyosis left deep inside the uterine muscle is still there and will continue to cause pain and bleeding. However, if the adenomyosis hasn't penetrated deeply into the uterine muscle, it is possible to get relief with an ablation. In women who are not ready to have a hysterectomy, pain can be reduced by taking NSAIDS during menstruation. These drugs inhibit prostaglandins that cause the uterus to contract and would thereby relieve some of the pain associated with this disorder. Other options for treatment include natural progesterone cream, use of a heating pad on the abdomen and herbal supplements. Hormonal suppression including using a continuous birth control pill may also be effective since this will stop menstrual cycles completely. Other options include implantation of a progesterone-releasing IUD, aromatase inhibitors, GnRH analogs, and uterine artery embolization.

All About Estrogen Dominance

Estrogen dominance refers to an imbalance of the estrogen and progesterone hormones in a woman's body. Typically, estrogen levels will remain in the normal range while progesterone levels will fall well below normal. This will cause a condition where unopposed estrogen is left in the body, and this can lead to all kinds of health problems with the most notable being an increased risk for breast cancer.

As I was doing research for this book, I discovered that adenomyosis has been linked to a condition called estrogen dominance. The more I learned about estrogen dominance, the more I suspected that I was affected by this disorder. Dr. John Lee was the actual physician who coined the term "estrogen dominance". It refers to a condition where there is insufficient progesterone in relation to estrogen in a woman's body. This intrigued me, so I went back and pulled out my old medical records to see what my progesterone levels were during the 17 years that I suffered from adenomyosis. To my surprise, I found that progesterone levels were never tested! The hormones that were tested were FSH, LH, prolactin, and estradiol.

I found out that Dr. Lee's office was in California and noticed that I could have my hormone levels checked by ordering a test through his website. I learned that a saliva test was a more accurate way to identify hormone imbalances than a blood test. I found this very interesting since all previous hormone tests done on me were by blood testing. I decided to go ahead with the saliva test which was ultimately tested by ZRT laboratories. The following are the results:

Estradiol	2.3	In range (normal is 1.3-3.3)
Progesterone	154	In range (normal is 75-270)
Ratio: Pg/E2	67	**Out of Range (normal is 100-500)**

Note: Pg stands for progesterone, E2 stands for estradiol

According to ZRT laboratories:
 "The Ratio: Pg/E2 on the third line of the report applies to women. This ratio, if either high or low, is a significant indicator of imbalance between estrogen and progesterone levels."
(www.zrtlab.com, 2012)

According to Labrix Clinical Services:
"Estrogen dominance is illustrated by a low Pg/E2 ratio." (Labrix Clinical Services, Inc., 2012)

As you can see, my Pg/E2 ratio is significantly low. This confirmed to me that I am, at least at the present time, estrogen dominant. I now strongly suspect that I have been estrogen dominant for most of my reproductive life due to my symptoms, and this condition may have been a major factor in the development of adenomyosis. This also could have played a role in other health issues such as allergies and failed spinal fusions which are discussed later in this book.

The causes of low progesterone include menopause, polycystic ovarian syndrome, exposure to xenoestrogens, exposure to synthetic progestins, poor diet, lack of exercise, certain medications and thyroid disorders.

The following are symptoms associated with estrogen dominance. This is not a comprehensive list but rather a list of some of the most common signs of this condition.

Allergies, asthma and sinus congestion
Cold hands and feet
Headaches (including migraines)
Depression and anxiety
Breast cancer
Endometrial cancer
Weight gain in the hips, thighs and abdomen
Fatigue
Insomnia
Foggy thinking
Hypoglycemia
Increased risk of blood clots
Mood swings
Irritability
Osteoporosis
Pre-menopausal bone loss
Polycystic ovarian syndrome
Decreased sex drive
Uterine fibroids

Fibrocystic breast disease
Endometriosis
Premenstrual syndrome
Irregular or heavy periods
Spotting between periods
Infertility
Bloating
Digestive problems
Dry eyes
Unwanted hair growth
Hair loss
Carbohydrate cravings
Magnesium and zinc deficiencies

The majority of the above symptoms are those that I had during my 17 year journey of suffering with adenomyosis. Interestingly, just in the last few years, I have begun to have a terrible time with cold hands and feet, especially at night. In fact, I currently go to bed with a heating pad on my feet. If I don't I can't sleep because my feet are ice cold. I am hoping that this will resolve with my use of progesterone cream which is discussed later in this book.

What are Xenoestrogens?

Xenoestrogens are synthetic (man made) estrogens that mimic the effects of estrogen found in the human body. They disrupt hormonal activity and can be extremely dangerous. There are around 70,000 chemicals known to disrupt hormonal levels in the human body. Below is a list of some more common xenoestrogens and where they are found in the environment. As you can see, some of these products have been banned from use.

PCBs - banned from use in 1979
PBBs - can be found in plastics
Pthalates - provides durability and flexibility to plastics
Petrochemicals - byproducts of oil and gasoline
Organochorides - dry cleaning products, chemicals used in the
                     bleaching of paper
BPAs - used in the lining of food and beverage cans

DDT - pesticide that was banned from use in 1972; however, this
chemical still exists in the environment to this day
Dioxins - released during pesticide manufacturing and combustion
processes
Endosulfans - insecticide
Atrazines - herbicide
Bisphenol A - food preservative
Parabens - lotions
Ethinyl estradiol - component of birth control pills

Some examples of specific products that contain xenoestrogens include the food coloring dye FD&C Red #3, paint fumes, nail polish, nail polish remover and household cleaners.

Diet and Estrogen Dominance

Diet plays a vital role in both the development and the treatment of estrogen dominance. In general, processed foods will exacerbate the condition, and fresh, organic foods will help to control it. The following are recommended foods for women with estrogen dominance:

Fiber - this nutrient helps to rid the body of excess estrogen by regulating bowel function. It feeds the normal flora in the gastrointestinal tract, and this in turn helps to metabolize hormones. If stool is retained in the colon due to constipation, the body will reabsorb the estrogen that it is trying to eliminate. Good sources of fiber include beans, nuts, seeds, oatmeal, and fresh vegetables.

Omega-3 fatty acids - In addition to reducing inflammation, omega-3 fatty acids have been shown to help the body balance hormone levels. An imbalance of omega-3 to omega-6 fatty acids in the diet has been shown to be a factor in estrogen dominance. Good sources include anchovies, mackerel, wild salmon, herring, sardines, tuna, walnuts, flaxseed, and canola, soybean and olive oils.

B vitamins - These nutrients help to balance hormone levels. Vitamin B6 specifically can help to increase progesterone production. Good sources include tuna, salmon, turkey, chicken, lentils, beans, potatoes, milk, bananas, pomegranate, avocado and eggs.

Flaxseed - In addition to high levels of omega 3 fatty acids, flaxseed contains the highest known source of lignans in any food. Lignans have been shown to inhibit enzymes that are involved in estrogen production. Flaxseed is also one of the best known sources of phytoestrogens.

Foods high in sulfur - These foods are known to help keep the liver healthy so it can rid the body of toxins and excess estrogen. Examples are onions, garlic, lemons, and leafy green vegetables.

Foods high in magnesium and zinc - These nutrients can help to increase progesterone production. They can be found in bran, dark chocolate, pumpkin, squash, flaxseed, sesame seeds, sunflower seeds, almonds, edamame, molasses, roast beef, oysters, wheat germ, peanuts, crab and lamb.

Organic foods - because of the way they are grown, organic foods contain less xenoestrogens thereby decreasing the amount of exposure to these dangerous substances.

Phytoestrogens - These substances have been shown to compete with estrogen receptor sites. They are weaker than estrogen found in the body thereby blocking the impact of more potent estrogens including xenoestrogens. Foods that contain this valuable nutrient include flaxseed (see above), sesame seeds, pistachios, sunflower seeds, almonds, beans, soy, fruits, vegetables, multigrain bread, rye and barley.

Cruciferous vegetables - These vegetables contain a substance called diindolylmethane that has been shown to help the body rid itself of excess estrogen. They include broccoli and cauliflower and are highly recommended for women with estrogen dominance.

Other foods that may help in women with estrogen dominance include wheat germ, kelp and walnuts.

Foods to avoid include caffeine, sugars, animal meats, processed dairy products, and other processed foods. A low carbohydrate and low fat diet are also advisable.

Yeast Infections and Estrogen Dominance

A discussion of the relationship between yeast infections and estrogen levels is also of note here. Estrogen is known to support the growth of Candida albicans, the microorganism responsible for vaginal yeast infections. Also, yeast infections are more commonly reported among women who are on birth control pills. In my case, I probably had estrogen dominance during those 17 years, and I was taking birth controls pills. This would clearly explain why I struggled with repeated vaginal yeast infections over the course of my reproductive years.

Headaches and Estrogen Dominance

Hormonal migraine headaches have been associated an imbalance of estrogen and progesterone hormone levels prior to a woman's menstrual period. It has been reported that approximately 60 percent of these headaches occur in women when progesterone levels are low. Birth control pills with high estrogen levels seem to be a trigger. It has also been noted that headaches seemed to improve with low dose estrogen birth control pills and didn't occur in women who used progesterone only birth control pills. Other ways to help combat these headaches include avoiding processed foods, simple sugars, and baked goods. NSAIDS have also been shown to help combat these headaches; however, NSAIDS in my case helped very little.

Breast Cancer and Estrogen Dominance

There has been much information about the role of estrogen in the development in breast cancer. However, recent studies have shown that progesterone also plays a role in the development of this type of cancer. Progesterone has been shown to inhibit both normal breast cell growth and the growth of breast cancer cells.

In order to fully understand the relationship between estrogen, progesterone and breast cancer, we must address how these hormones function in the life of cells. All cells have a finite life span. Apoptosis means the end of the life of the cell (cell death). The apoptosis aspect of this system must work well; otherwise, cells would grow out of control. This out-of-control growth is called cancer.

There are many different genes in the human genome. We will be talking about two specific genes in this section, the BCl 2 gene and the p53 gene. When the BCl 2 gene is stimulated by estrogen, cells divide, proliferate and prevent cell death (apoptosis). However, the p53 gene is involved in apoptosis and is stimulated by progesterone. When these hormones are in balance, the system works well. However, when these two hormones are out of balance, as in the case of estrogen dominance, things can go very wrong. If the estrogen is stimulating the BC1 2 gene and causing division and proliferation and there is not enough progesterone to cause the cells to cycle into apoptosis, cells can grow out of control, possibly leading to breast cancer.

Interestingly, the use of synthetic (man made) progesterone does not upregulate the p53 gene. This means that the use of synthetic progesterone is not protective against breast cancer since it is unable to activate the gene necessary for apoptosis. Therefore, synthetic progesterone cannot be substituted for human progesterone or a bioidentical progesterone for protection against breast cancer in estrogen dominant women.

The following is an excerpt from a non-copyrighted article written by Virginia Hopkins (2012). It clearly shows the link between estrogen dominance and breast cancer.

1) The earliest clinical study that we know of on progesterone and breast cancer was done at Johns Hopkins University back in 1981 (Cowan et al, American Journal of Epidemiology). They measured estrogen and progesterone in a group of women, then divided them into two groups: those with normal progesterone levels and those with low progesterone levels. They followed these women for 20 years and found that in the women with low progesterone, the incidence of breast cancer was over 80 percent greater than those with normal progesterone, and the incidence of all cancers was ten times higher than in women with normal progesterone.

2) In 1996, researchers measured women's progesterone before breast cancer surgery and found that those with normal progesterone levels had an 18 year survival rate - twice that of women with low progesterone at the time of surgery. (Mohr et al, British Journal of Cancer).

3) Three studies in particular have shown progesterone's effect on breast cells. One, by Foidart et al and published in the journal Fertility and Sterility in 1998 concluded, "Exposure to progesterone for 14 days reduced the estradiol-induced proliferation of normal breast epithelial cells in vivo." Another, by Malet et al and published in the Journal of Steroid Biochemistry and Molecular Biology, in 2000 concluded, "Cells exhibited a proliferative appearance after E2 [estradiol] treatment, and returned to a quiescent appearance when P[rogesterone] was added to E2. P[rogesterone] appear(s) predominantly to inhibit cell growth, both in the presence and absence of E2.

The third study tested the effects of transdermal (rubbed into the skin) hormones in healthy young women planning to undergo minor breast surgery for aesthetic reasons or for benign breast disease. Ten to 13 days before surgery, four groups of women applied either estradiol cream, progesterone cream, a combination of estradiol and progesterone, or a placebo cream (with no hormones in it). At surgery, biopsies were done to measure estrogen and progesterone levels, and the level of cell proliferation rates. (A high level of cell proliferation is a marker for breast cancer.) The study demonstrated that both hormones were well absorbed through the skin into the breast tissue. But even more significant, estradiol increased cell proliferation by 230 percent, whereas progesterone decreased it by more than 400 percent. The estradiol-progesterone combination maintained the normal proliferation rate. (Chang et al, Fertility and Sterility)

In a study done by Formby and Wiley and published in the Annals of Clinical and Laboratory Science (1998) showed a 90% cell death rate of T47-D breast cancer cells when exposed to 10 microM progesterone for 72 hours. This study also reports that after 24 hours exposure to progesterone, the BCl 2 gene was found to be downregulated and the p53 was upregulated.

According to the authors, "progesterone at a concentration similar to that seen during the third trimester of pregnancy exhibited a strong antiproliferative effect on at least two breast cancer cell lines. Apoptosis was induced in the progesterone receptor expressing T47-D breast cancer cells." (Formby &Wiley, 1998)

These studies strongly demonstrate the role of progesterone in breast health. This new information shows that not only unopposed estrogen but also low progesterone plays roles in the development of breast cancer. It is vitally important to look at the levels of both of these hormones to determine a possible hormone imbalance that might predispose women to breast cancer.

Progesterone and Bone Health

Recent studies have shown that progesterone helps to promote new bone growth by stimulating osteoblast differentiation. Low progesterone levels have been linked to lower levels of osteoblasts that are needed to rebuild bone. As a result, this leads to bones that are weak and brittle. It is reported that progesterone stimulates new bone formation while estradiol inhibits bone resorption. Molecular studies using polymerase chain reaction (PCR) have shown that progesterone has action in bone formation. According to a study by MacNamara, O'Shaughnessy, Manduca and Loughrey (1995), "The finding that [progesterone] is expressed at both the level of mRNA and protein in several osteoblast-like cell lines as well as in human primary osteoblast cultures indicates that bone-forming osteoblast cells are direct targets for progesterone action."

Several studies have shown that progesterone does indeed play a role in promoting bone health. According to Dr. John Lee, M.D. (2012), after treating his patients with a transdermal progesterone cream for three years, he identified a 15% improvement in bone mineral density even though there was no estrogen supplementation. In a study by Seifert-Klauss and Prior and published in the Journal of Osteoporosis (2010), the researchers reported that progesterone and anti-resorptive drugs in combination increase bone mineral density and increase bone formation.

Since progesterone appears to play a critical role in bone health, I became very suspicious that the cause of my failed spinal fusions may be directly linked to estrogen dominance. According to the study by Seifert-Klauss and Prior (2010), "Subclinical ovulatory disturbances may pose a risk for bone remodeling imbalance and bone loss despite regular, estrogen-sufficient menstrual cycles." In my case, I did have regular 28 day cycles. In addition, during the few times over the 17 years that I had my hormones tested, my estrogen levels always came back normal. But I now know that I did have adenomyosis that could have been caused by low progesterone levels. Also according to Seifert-Klauss and Prior (2010), "The fact that bone morphogenic proteins play a crucial role in both ovulation and bone metabolism points towards a functional link between bone and reproductive systems...." It is interesting to note that in addition to the low progesterone levels, the third fusion finally succeeded with the use of synthetic bone morphogenic protein during surgery. Of particular interest in Seifert-Klauss and Prior's report (2010) was "Medoxyprogesterone increases pre-menopausal spine bone mineral density as physiological-dose cyclic therapy in a randomized controlled trial for healthy women experiencing hypothalamic amenorrhea, oligomenorrhea, anovulation or short luteal phase cycles." Considering the abnormal Pg/E2 ratio, infertility issues, and failed spinal fusions, it appears to me that estrogen dominance may have played not only a critical role in adenomyosis but also could have been a major player in the failed spinal fusions.

Conclusion

Adenomyosis is very difficult to diagnose. A hysterectomy will completely stop the symptoms; however, many women with this condition are too young to consider this option. More studies need to be done to determine more effective treatments for women who still want to have children. Other conditions of the uterus cause symptoms that are similar to adenomyosis. Some of these include fibroids, endometriosis and endometrial polyps. In fact, this disorder of the uterus often occurs in conjunction with fibroids or endometriosis. I believe that physicians need to be more educated on this disorder and listen closely to their patients and their particular symptoms. Paying close attention to the subtle differences in symptomatology among all of these uterine disorders may just prevent someone else from enduring years of misdiagnosed conditions and anxiety.

In doing research for this book, I was amazed at how all of the pieces of the puzzle came together when learning about estrogen dominance. Although a lot of this cannot be proven, I wonder how much of not only my health issues but also health problems in my family could be possibly linked back to estrogen dominance.

The fact that my maternal grandmother died from breast cancer at a very young age makes me wonder if she also had a hormonal imbalance such as estrogen dominance. My grandfather worked in the oil business, and he and my grandmother lived near an oil well for one year after she gave birth to her first child. If she was estrogen dominant and was exposed to high levels of xenoestrogens, this could possibly explain the development of her breast cancer. Of course, the cancer could have also been due to the exposure of xenoestrogens alone or something different altogether, but it does make me think and wonder.

In the 1980's, my mother struggled with similar menstrual difficulties as I had been through, and she also ended up having a hysterectomy. She was told that she had fibroid tumors. However, this was 30 years ago, and we now know that adenomyosis and fibroids have similar symptoms. Did she actually suffer from adenomyosis too? Maybe so.

I suffered almost my whole life with terrible allergies. Both my mother and my maternal grandmother also suffered with these problems. I specifically have "flares" in sinus congestion during PMS. Additionally, my maternal grandmother had asthma. Allergies and asthma are known signs for estrogen dominance. Could this all be linked?

And then there is the issue of my failed spinal fusions. I did not have any risk factors for this surgery, such as smoking, and my physicians were baffled by the failure of my bones to fuse. When I realized that I might be estrogen dominant and learned that progesterone was vitally important in bone health, this made me strongly suspect that the lack of necessary progesterone in my body was playing a role in these failed spinal fusions.

It is interesting in my case to compare the different birth control pills that were prescribed over the 17 years. As you can see below, the birth control pills that I was prescribed earlier in my treatment were higher in estrogen and lower in progesterone than those prescribed later in my treatment. In reviewing my story, it can be seen that my symptoms were generally better in the later years at a time when I was taking pills that were lower in estrogen and higher in progesterone.

Ortho Tri Cyclen (norgestimate/ethinyl estradiol)	.035 mg	.18, .215, .25 mg
Ortho Novum 7/7/7 (norethindrone/ethinyl estradiol)	.035 mg	.5, .75, 1 mg
Lo Estrin (norethindrone acetate/ ethinyl estradiol)	:02 mg	1.0 mg
Yasmin (drospirenone/ethinyl estradiol)	.03 mg	3.0 mg

My symptoms also improved with changes in diet. As discussed earlier, I went from a diet high in processed foods to one high in fruits and vegetables. I particularly liked salads and ate quite a bit of broccoli and cauliflower. These cruciferous vegetables contain diindolylmethane which helps the body to rid itself of excess estrogen. In addition, I began to sprinkle flaxseed on my meals whenever possible. It is very interesting to note that omega-3 fatty acids found in flaxseed have been shown to help balance hormone levels. Specifically, flaxseed contains lignans that inhibit enzymes involved in estrogen production. Finally the phytoestrogens found in fruits and vegetables compete with estrogen receptor sites in the body. They are weaker estrogens and block the actions of more potent estrogens.

Considering all of this information, it seems clear to me why my symptoms improved when I changed my diet.

Although adenomyosis is a benign condition, it can severely affect a person's lifestyle due to the pain and blood loss. As you will see from my story, the diagnosis in my case took about 17 years, and during that time, I was also diagnosed with endometriosis and an endometrial polyp. Additional research is so important to learn more about this disorder of the uterus. Also, new and improved imaging needs to be developed to help identify adenomyosis, especially with diffuse involvement.

Estrogen dominance is sadly not easily accepted by western physicians. However, with my experience, I do strongly believe that this is a very real hormonal problem in women that can lead to debilitating conditions. I also suggest a Pg/E2 ratio should be included with all female hormone testing to identify hormonal imbalances that could lead to other more serious and even deadly diseases.

It is my intention with this book to bring adenomyosis and estrogen dominance some much needed attention. Hopefully in the future, scientists will find a better way to detect and treat this condition. Finally, I hope physicians and researchers look more deeply into estrogen dominance and realize the critical importance of a healthy balance between estrogen and progesterone levels in women's health.

References

Bayer. (2012). *Yasmin.* Retrieved November 30, 2012, from http://www.yasmin-us.com

Balanced Concepts. (2012). *List of Xenoestrogens - Chemical Estrogens.* Retrieved December 9, 2012, from http://www.balancedconcepts.net/tips_avoid_xenoestrogens.pdf

Body Ecology. (2012). *PMS and Candida Overgrowth: The Dangers of Estrogen Dominance.* Retrieved December 6, 2012, from http://bodyecology.com/articles/pms-and-candida-overgrowth

Boomsma, Diane RPh. And Paoletti, Jim RPh. (2002) *A Review of Current Research on the Effects of Progesterone.* International Journal of Pharmaceutical Compounding, Vol. 6, No. 4. Retrieved December 2, 2012, from http://hemingways.org/GIDinfo/drugdata/progest_review.pdf

Drugs.com. (2012). *Bentyl.* Retrieved December 8, 2012, from http://www.drugs.com/cdi/bentyl.html

Drugs.com. (2012). *Levsin.* Retrieved November 29, 2012, from http://www.drugs.com/cdi/levsin.html

Drugs.com. (2012). *Ponstel.* Retrieved November 30, 2012, from http://www.drugs.com/cdi/ponstel.html

Drugs.com. (2012). *Prilosec.* Retrieved December 8, 2012, from http://www.drugs.com/prilosec.html

Formby, B. and Wiley, T.S. (1999). *BCL2, survivin and variant DC44v7-v10 are downregulated and p53 is upregulated in breast cancer cells by progesterone: Inhibition of cell growth and induction of apoptosis.* Mol Cell Biochem 202 (1-2). Retrieved December 8, 2012, from http://www.ncbi.nlm.nih.gov/pubmed/10705995

Formby, B & Wiley, T.S. (1998). *Progesterone Inhibits Growth and Induces Apoptosis in Breast Cancer Cells: Inverse Effects on BCl-2 and p53.* Ann Clin Lab Sci Vol. 28 no. 6. Retrieved December 9, 2012, from http://annclinlabsci.org/content/28/6/360.abstract

Hopkins, Virginia. (2011). *Dr. Ellen Grant, Lynne McTaggart and WDDTY Newsletter Launch Muddled Personal Attack on Dr. John Lee and on Natural Progesterone.* Retrieved December 6, 2012, from http://www.johnleemd.com/store/pgattack/html

Kim, Ben M.D. (2012). *Estrogen Dominance: Is It Affecting Your Health?* Retrieved November 30, 2012, from http://drbenkim.com/estrogen-dominance-health.htm

Labrix Clinical Services, Inc. (2011). *Hormones of Relativity: The Pg/E2 ratio and estrogen dominance.* Retrieved January 15, 2013, from http://archive.aweber.com/saliva-testing

Lee, John M.D. (2012). *Osteoporosis Treatment During or Shortly After Menopause.* Retrieved December 8, 2012, from http://www.johnleemd.com/store/osteoporosis.html

Livestrong.com. (2011). *Foods That Contain Phytoestrogen.* Retrieved December 6, 2012, from http://www.livestrong.com/article/83849-foods-contain-phytoestrogens

Livestrong.com. (2011). *Foods That Lower High Estrogen.* Retrieved December 6, 2012, from http://www.livestrong.com/article/482045-foods-that-lower-high-estrogen

Livestrong.com. (2011). *Headaches and Low Progesterone.* Retrieved January 6, 2013, from http://www.livestrong.com/article/496077-headaches-low-progesterone

Livestrong.com. (2011). *How Does Clomid Work?* Retrieved November 30, 2012, from http://www.livestrong.com/article/33273-clomid-work

Livestrong.com. (2011). *What Foods Reduce Estrogen Dominance?* Retrieved December 6, 2012, from http://www.livestrong.com/article/16099-foods-reduce-estrogen

MacNamara, P., O'Shaughnessy, C., Manduca, P., Loughrey, H.C. *Progesterone Receptors are Expressed in Human Osteoblast-Like Cell Lines and in Primary Human Osteoblast Cultures.* Calcified Tissue International 57(6). Retrieved December 2, 2012, from http://link.springer.com/article

Mayo Clinic. (2012). *Adenomyosis.* Retrieved November 27, 2012, from http://www.mayoclinic.com/health/Adenomyosis

Mayo Clinic. (2012). *Endometrial Ablation.* Retrieved October 19, 2012, from http://www.mayoclinic.com/health/endometrial-ablation

Mayo Clinic. (2012). *Uterine Polyps.* Retrieved December 9, 2012, from http://www.mayoclinic.com/health/uterine-polyps

Mills, Dixie M.D. (2011). *What is estrogen dominance? (It's probably not what you think!).* Retrieved November 30, 2012, from http://www.womentowomen.com/menopause/estrogendominance

Northrup, Christiane M.D. (2012). *Estrogen Dominance.* Retrieved November 30, 2012, from http://www.drnorthrup.com/womenshealth/healthcenter

PubMed Health. (2010). *Adenomyosis.* Retrieved November 27, 2012, from http://www.ncbi.nlm.nih.gov

PubMed Health. (2012). *Clomiphene.* Retrieved November 30, 2012, from http://www.ncbi.nlm.nih.gov/pubmedhealth

PubMed Health. (2011). *Endometriosis.* Retrieved January 6, 2013, from http://www.ncbi.nlm.nih.gov/pubmedhealth

PubMed Health. (2012) *Fibrocystic Breast Disease.* Retrieved January 6, 2012, from http://www.ncbi.nlm.nih.gov/pubmedhealth

PubMed Health. (2012). *Fluoxetine.* Retrieved December 4, 2012, from http://www.ncbi.nlm.nih.gov/pubmedhealth

PubMed Health. (2012). *Hyoscyamine.* Retrieved November 29, 2012 from http://www.ncbi.nlm.nih.gov/pubmedhealth

PubMed Health. (2011). *Irritable Bowel Syndrome.* Retrieved January 15, 2013, from http://www.ncbi.nlm.nih.gov/pubmedhealth/PMH0001292

PubMed Health. (2012). *Mefenamic Acid.* Retrieved November 30, 2012, from http://www.ncbi.nlm.nih.gov/pubmedhealth

PubMed Health. (2010). *Premenstrual Dysphoric Disorder.* Retrieved November 30, 2012, from http://www.ncbi.nlm.nih.gov/pubmedhealth

PubMed Health. (2012). *Sumatriptan Oral and Nasal.* Retrieved December 4, 2012, from http://www.ncbi.nlm.nih.gov/pubmedhealth

RadiologyInfo.org. (2012). *Sonohysterography.* Retrieved December 8, 2012, from http://www.radiologyinfo.org/en/info.cfm?pg=hysterosono

Redwine, David B. (2012). *Adenomyosis: A Common Cause of Uterine Symptoms after Age 30.* Retrieved November 27, 2012, from http://www.endometriosissurgeon.com

Seifert-Klauss, Vanadin & Prior, Jerilynn C. (2010). *Progesterone and Bone: Actions Promoting Bone Health in Women.* J Osteoporos: 845180. Retrieved January 6, 2012, from http://www.hindawi.com/journals/josteo

Simon, Carolyn N.D. (2012). *The Hormone Effect - Every Woman's Health Issue.* Retrieved December 6, 2012, from http://www.healthpost.co.nz/the-hormone-effect-every-   woman's-health-issue

Stoppler, Melissa M.D. (2012). *Uterine Fibroids.* www.medicinenet.com. Retrieved January 6, 2013, from http://www.medicinenet.com/uterine-fibroids

WebMD. (2012). *50+: Live Better, Longer.* Retrieved December 4, 2012, from http://www.webmd.com/healthy-aging/omega-3-fatty-acid-facts

WebMD. (2012). *What is Adenomyosis?* Retrieved November 27, 2012, from http://women.webmd.com/adenomyosis

WebMD. (2012). *Endometrial Ablation.* Retrieved October 19, 2012, from http://women.webmd.com/endometrial-ablation

WebMD. (2012). *Migraines, Headaches and Hormones.* Retrieved December 6, 2012, from http://www.webmd.com/migraines-headaches/guide.hormones

Wikipedia. (2012). *Adenomyosis.* Retrieved November 27, 2012, from http://en.wikipedia.org/wiki/Adenomyosis

Wikipedia. (2012). *Bicornuate Uterus.* Retrieved November 29, 2012, from http://en.wikipedia.org/wiki/Bicornuate_uterus

Wikipedia. (2012). *Retroverted Uterus.* Retrieved October 19, 2012, from http://en.wikipedia.org/wiki/Retroverted_uterus

Wikipedia. (2012). *Stenosis of Uterine Cervix.* Retrieved November 30, 2012, from http://en.wikipedia.org/wiki/Stenosis_of_uterine_cervix

Wikipedia. (2012). *Xenoestrogen.* Retrieved December 5, 2012, from http://en.wikipedia.org/wiki/Xenoestrogen

ZRT lab. (2004). *Understanding Your Test Results.* Retrieved January 15, 2013, from http://www.canaryclub.org/canaryclub/docs

www.ingramcontent.com/pod-product-compliance
Lightning Source LLC
Chambersburg PA
CBHW080832180526

45168CB00006B/2657